ACUPUNCTURE BENEFITS AND TECHNIQUES

A Comprehensive Guide to Acupuncture's Healing Power and Techniques for Enhanced Well-being

WILFREDO CARSON

INTRODUCTION

Acupuncture, an ancient medical treatment based on traditional Chinese medicine (TCM), has acquired a worldwide reputation for its comprehensive approach to health and well-being. This treatment includes inserting small needles into certain places on the body to increase energy flow and restore equilibrium. As we go into the depths of acupuncture, this research seeks to explain its complexities, from historical evolution to present uses. The goal of this book is to provide a full understanding of acupuncture, including its tremendous advantages and the procedures used by practitioners. In doing so, we hope to bridge the gap between traditional wisdom and modern science, providing insights into the significance of understanding acupuncture for both practitioners and the general public.

THE PURPOSE OF THE BOOK

The fundamental goal of this book is to explain the numerous benefits of acupuncture, which range from its physiological effects to its impact on mental and emotional well-being. Acupuncture is more than just a supplemental therapy; it has grown into a freestanding medical profession with a diverse range of uses. A detailed examination of its mechanics and effects will provide readers with a profound knowledge of why acupuncture has survived for centuries and continues to thrive in today's healthcare scene. By delving into the goal of acupuncture, we hope to provide practitioners, academics, and interested readers with a comprehensive resource that goes beyond surface-level explanations and explores the depths of its therapeutic potential.

A BRIEF HISTORY OF ACUPUNCTURE

To understand the core of acupuncture, one must journey through the history of traditional Chinese medicine. Acupuncture dates back over 2,500 years and is based on old philosophical principles such as Yin and Yang and the flow of Qi (energy). Acupuncture was first recorded in the Huangdi Neijing (Yellow Emperor's Inner Canon), a fundamental literature that provided the groundwork for Traditional Chinese Medicine. Acupuncture has progressed over the years from simple stone needles to the tiny, metallic needles we use today. This journey combines Taoist philosophy, Confucianism, and practical observations, resulting in a holistic treatment method that sees the body as an interconnected network of energy paths.

Exploring acupuncture's historical context not only sheds light on its cultural significance but also lays the groundwork for comprehending its relevance in modern healthcare practices.

<u>Importance of Understanding Acupuncture</u>

Understanding the origins and principles of acupuncture is becoming increasingly important in today's quickly changing medical scene. As traditional and alternative medicine combine, acupuncture's value is becoming more widely recognized. From pain management to stress reduction, acupuncture provides a comprehensive approach that is consistent with the current emphasis on patient-centered care. Furthermore, as research into the physiological mechanisms underlying acupuncture continues, the relevance of comprehending its principles becomes increasingly clear. The integration of acupuncture into mainstream healthcare necessitates a shared understanding among healthcare professionals and the general population. This section discusses the importance of understanding acupuncture not only from a historical and cultural perspective but also in terms of its potential to influence the future of healthcare.

Concepts of Acupuncture

Acupuncture is based on a set of core beliefs that define its practice and consequences. These beliefs, based on ancient Chinese philosophy, serve as the theoretical underpinning for acupuncturists' healing practices. Qi, often known as vital energy, is a key concept in acupuncture. TCM believes that the balance and movement of Qi through meridians affects physical, mental, and emotional well-being. Acupuncture sites, where needles are put, are precisely placed to control Qi flow and restore balance to the body's systems. Meridians, the routes via which Qi circulates, comprise a complex network that connects many organs and tissues. The concept of Yin and Yang, which represent opposing yet complementary forces, underpins the equilibrium sought in acupuncture treatments.

Another fundamental notion in acupuncture is the Five Elements hypothesis, which associates specific organs and meridians with the elements wood, fire, earth, metal, and water. This comprehensive approach allows acupuncturists to resolve imbalances and disharmonies by taking into account how various aspects interact within the body. Traditional acupuncture diagnostic procedures such as pulse and tongue diagnosis provide additional information about the state of the body's Qi and general health.

<u>Techniques for Acupuncture</u>

Acupuncture treatments include a variety of modalities, each designed to address a unique health condition. The most popular approach is to place small needles into acupuncture points, with varying depths and manipulations. Another approach for increasing Qi flow and warming the body is moxibustion, which involves burning mugwort over acupuncture sites.

Cupping includes placing cups on the skin to create suction, which promotes blood circulation and relieves muscle tension. Acupressure is a non-invasive treatment that includes applying pressure to acupuncture points with fingers or specialized equipment. Electroacupuncture, a recent innovation, involves the use of electric currents in acupuncture needles to increase stimulation.

Auriculotherapy, which treats the ear as a microsystem that reflects the entire body, is another specialist method. Laser acupuncture, a non-invasive technique utilizing low-level lasers, is gaining popularity due to its precision and efficacy. Scalp acupuncture, a technique established in the 1970s, focuses on certain locations of the scalp that correspond to various parts of the body. Understanding these strategies enables practitioners to personalize treatments to specific requirements and situations, enhancing the therapeutic effects of acupuncture.

Clinical Applications of Acupuncture

Acupuncture's adaptability extends to a wide range of clinical uses, making it an invaluable instrument in the hands of healthcare practitioners. Pain management is one of the most extensively researched and well-acknowledged applications of acupuncture. Acupuncture is effective in treating chronic back pain and migraines by regulating the body's pain-signaling pathways. Acupuncture's anti-inflammatory actions lead to its effectiveness in treating a variety of inflammatory disorders.

Acupuncture is useful for managing mental health issues in addition to pain management. Acupuncture effectively treats anxiety, sadness, and stress-related problems by inducing relaxation and harmonizing neurotransmitter levels. Acupuncture's effect on the autonomic nerve and endocrine systems leads to its success in treating stress-related illnesses.

Acupuncture is also used to treat fertility and reproductive health issues. Acupuncture has been used in fertility treatments and to support women undergoing assisted reproductive technologies because it regulates hormonal balance and improves blood supply to reproductive organs. Acupuncture has also shown promise in addressing menopausal symptoms like hot flashes and sleep difficulties.

Acupuncture's influence extends to digestive health, with treatments aimed at gastrointestinal diseases like irritable bowel syndrome (IBS) and acid reflux. Acupuncture's ability to control digestive functions and reduce inflammation helps it succeed in this field. Respiratory disorders, dermatological issues, and immune system modulation expand the clinical applications of acupuncture.

Research and Evidence-Based Practices

As acupuncture obtains acceptance in mainstream medicine, a growing body of research is devoted to understanding its mechanics and developing evidence-based procedures. Acupuncture's efficacy in various disorders has been investigated in rigorous clinical trials and systematic reviews, which have contributed to its inclusion in treatment guidelines for certain ailments.

Neuroimaging studies have revealed the neurological underpinnings underlying acupuncture, including its impact on brain activity, neurotransmitter release, and pain regulation. Furthermore, research has provided insight into acupuncture's effects on inflammation, immunological function, and endorphin release, providing a scientific foundation for its therapeutic benefits.

However, standardizing acupuncture protocols remains difficult due to the customized character of treatments and the variety of modalities used. The placebo effect, which is frequently noted as a potential confounder in acupuncture research, demands rigorous study design and control procedures. Despite these obstacles, a growing amount of research supports the integration of acupuncture into evidence-based healthcare procedures, enabling collaboration between traditional and modern medical treatments.

Acupuncture is a powerful monument to the lasting wisdom of traditional Chinese medicine, effortlessly combining old philosophy with modern scientific understanding. The goal of this book has been to peel back the layers of acupuncture, investigate its historical foundations, delve into its essential concepts, and explain the various procedures used by practitioners. Understanding acupuncture is more than just an intellectual study; it is the key to unlocking its enormous potential for improving human health and well-being.

The historical voyage of acupuncture's history emphasizes its adaptability and durability, while the examination of essential concepts gives a theoretical framework for its application. Recognizing the significance of acupuncture in the modern healthcare landscape highlights its function as a helpful supplement to mainstream therapy. From the precise balance of Qi to the many procedures used, acupuncture provides a holistic approach to treatment that is applicable across a wide range of therapeutic applications.

As research advances and evidence-based methods emerge, acupuncture's incorporation into mainstream healthcare grows stronger.

The intersection of traditional knowledge and modern science ushers in a new era of collaborative and integrative medicine. Acupuncture, with its rich history and expanding clinical uses, urges practitioners, researchers, and curious readers to embrace its transformative potential for promoting health and harmony.

CHAPTER 1
THE FUNDAMENTALS OF ACUPUNCTURE

Acupuncture, a key component of traditional Chinese medicine (TCM), is a treatment that has roots in ancient Chinese philosophy and medical traditions. The term "acupuncture" comes from the Latin words "acus" (needle) and "pungent" (prick). The insertion of small needles into certain spots on the body is intended to restore the balance of vital energy, known as Qi, and enhance overall well-being. Acupuncture has a 2,500-year history and is based on the ancient Chinese notion that the body's vital energy runs along certain routes or meridians.

Definition & Origins

Acupuncture, as defined in modern medical contexts, is a therapeutic practice that includes inserting small needles into specific places on the body, known as acupuncture sites or acupoints. These acupoints are thought to be connected by meridians, which are energy channels that run throughout the body.

The practice began in ancient China, and its fundamental ideas are strongly founded in the

Chinese philosophy of balancing the opposing energies of Yin and Yang, as well as the harmony of Qi within the body.

Principles of Traditional Chinese Medicine

To truly grasp acupuncture, one must first study the principles of Traditional Chinese Medicine (TCM), which serve as the theoretical framework for this ancient healing practice. TCM sees the body as a holistic system with physical, mental, and spiritual components that are interrelated. The underlying principle of TCM is the balance of vital energy, or Qi, which circulates throughout the body via specialized paths known as meridians.

The harmonious flow of Qi is regarded as critical for preserving health, whereas abnormalities can lead to sickness. TCM also emphasizes organ interconnectivity and the impact of environmental factors such as climate and lifestyle on health.

<u>Qi and meridians</u>

Qi, often known as vital energy or life force, is important to understanding acupuncture. Qi circulates throughout the body, replenishing organs, tissues, and cells, and is essential for maintaining health and vitality.

According to TCM, interruptions in the flow of Qi can cause a variety of health problems.

The meridian system, which consists of 12 basic meridians and eight exceptional vessels, provides paths for Qi to flow. Each meridian is connected with a certain organ system and has distinct acupoints along its path. The expert placement of needles into these acupoints is said to regulate the flow of Qi, restoring balance and facilitating healing.

<u>Yin and Yang in Acupuncture.</u>

Acupuncture technique is inextricably linked to the notions of yin and Yang, which are central to Chinese philosophy. These opposing forces symbolize the dual aspect of existence, with Yin representing darkness, passivity, and cold, and Yang representing light, activity, and warmth. In acupuncture, health is defined as a dynamic equilibrium of Yin and Yang.

The meridians and organs of the body are classified as Yin or Yang, and disruptions in this equilibrium are thought to cause disease. Acupuncture seeks to restore harmony by altering the flow of Qi and modifying the Yin-Yang balance. Practitioners carefully choose acupuncture points and procedures based on the nature of the imbalance, attempting to restore balance to the body.

Acupuncture is based on ancient Chinese philosophy and Traditional Chinese Medicine concepts. The technique centers on the manipulation of Qi, the vital energy that flows through meridians, to restore balance and promote health. Understanding the connection of Yin and Yang is critical for treating imbalances and promoting overall well-being with acupuncture. Acupuncture, as a therapeutic intervention, is still being studied scientifically and clinically, providing a unique viewpoint on health and healing that crosses cultural barriers.

CHAPTER 2
ACUPUNCTURE TECHNIQUES

Traditional needle acupuncture is a key component of traditional Chinese medicine (TCM), including the insertion of tiny needles into precise spots on the body to control the flow of qi or vital energy. This technique relies heavily on needle insertion and manipulation. Practitioners use manipulation techniques such as twisting, lifting, and thrusting to precisely implant needles at certain places. Depth and angle are painstakingly tuned to target certain meridians and health concerns. Filiform, intradermal, and three-edged needles are among the various varieties employed in the therapy process, each serving a specific purpose. This traditional method of acupuncture has a long history, with roots in ancient Chinese philosophy and holistic healing ideas.

Modern Acupuncture Techniques: Acupuncture techniques have changed, adopting novel strategies to improve effectiveness and adapt to a wide range of patient needs. Electroacupuncture uses electrical stimulation on traditional acupuncture points to enhance the therapeutic effects. This approach is thought to increase the flow of energy and encourage endorphin production. Laser acupuncture is a non-invasive variant that uses low-intensity lasers rather than needles. This method is especially appealing to those who are opposed to traditional needle insertion because it provides a painless alternative while still targeting acupuncture sites.

Auricular acupuncture stimulates particular spots on the ear that reflect the complete body's architecture.

This modern adaption acknowledges the interdependence of numerous body parts and systems, resulting in a focused and holistic approach to treatment.

Acupressure and Meridian Massage are non-invasive alternatives to traditional needle acupuncture. Acupressure is the process of applying pressure to certain spots on the body, similar to acupuncture points, with the use of fingers, palms, or other equipment.

The manipulation of these pressure points is thought to stimulate the flow of qi and correct imbalances in the body. Kneading, rubbing, and tapping are all techniques that can be used to successfully stimulate these spots.

Acupressure provides numerous benefits, including pain alleviation and stress reduction. Meridian massage, on the other hand, focuses on the entire meridian system by applying massage methods to the body's energy lines. This method promotes relaxation and addresses meridian obstructions, resulting in overall well-being and equilibrium.

Moxibustion and Cupping: Moxibustion therapy is a component of traditional Chinese medicine that involves the burning of mugwort (Artemisia vulgaris) to stimulate certain acupuncture sites. This therapeutic practice attempts to improve the flow of qi and blood while treating a variety of health issues. The practitioner may utilize either direct or indirect moxibustion, depending on the patient's needs and the type of ailment being treated.

Cupping therapy is another ancient practice that involves placing cups on the skin to create a vacuum, which promotes blood flow and reduces tension. This procedure results in unique circular imprints on the skin, signaling the release of stagnant energy and poisons. Cupping is used to treat muscle discomfort, and respiratory difficulties, and improve general circulation.

Acupuncture techniques include a wide range of modalities, each with its ideas and applications. Traditional needle acupuncture, which is profoundly based on Chinese philosophy, focuses on exact needle insertion, manipulation, and the use of multiple needle kinds. Modern acupuncture techniques, such as electroacupuncture, laser acupuncture, and auricular acupuncture, provide unique solutions tailored to individual needs. Acupressure and meridian massage are non-invasive treatments that focus on pressure points and energy pathways to promote overall well-being. Moxibustion and cupping are traditional Chinese medical techniques that use heat and suction to stimulate specific areas, increasing the flow of qi and resolving a variety of health issues. The diverse range of acupuncture treatments illustrates the adaptability and continuous progress of this ancient healing art.

CHAPTER 3
HEALTH BENEFITS OF ACUPUNCTURE

Acupuncture, an ancient Chinese medical practice, has gained global recognition for its numerous health advantages. Its efficacy spans multiple domains, adding to people's overall well-being. One significant part of its medicinal promise is pain management. Acupuncture has been very effective in treating chronic pain, bringing comfort to people suffering from arthritis, fibromyalgia, and neuropathy. The intentional insertion of small needles at certain locations on the body causes the production of endorphins, the body's natural painkillers, resulting in pain relief and better mobility.

Musculoskeletal pain, which includes concerns such as back pain and joint abnormalities, is another area where acupuncture has demonstrated great benefit. By focusing on certain acupuncture points connected with the musculoskeletal system, this traditional treatment helps to reduce inflammation, promote blood circulation, and boost the body's natural healing mechanisms. Furthermore, acupuncture has shown efficacy in treating headaches and migraines, providing a non-pharmacological option for people seeking relief from these distressing disorders.

Acupuncture is beneficial not only for pain management but also for stress reduction and mental health. As a complementary therapy, acupuncture has been used to treat anxiety and depression, both of which are common in today's society. The insertion of needles regulates the body's stress response, which promotes relaxation and emotional well-being. Acupuncture has also been shown to alleviate insomnia, a typical expression of stress, by addressing underlying imbalances in the body's energy flow, resulting in healthier sleep patterns. Furthermore, acupuncture has shown potential in treating post-traumatic stress disorder (PTSD), offering a comprehensive approach to mental health care.

The complex relationship between acupuncture and the immune system reveals another aspect of its health advantages. Acupuncture increases the creation of immune cells, which strengthens the body's defenses against infections and disorders. This immune system support is especially important in the context of allergies and respiratory problems. Acupuncture has been studied as a complementary strategy to treating allergic reactions and improving respiratory function, demonstrating its potential as a comprehensive therapy for those with weakened immune and respiratory systems.

Women's health is a specific field in which acupuncture has shown significant advantages. Fertility, a common worry for many couples, has been treated with acupuncture by boosting hormonal balance and improving reproductive organ function. Menstrual abnormalities, ranging from irregular cycles to severe cramps, have also improved with acupuncture treatments, which offer a non-invasive and drug-free way to manage these problems. Acupuncture has also been used as a supportive therapy throughout pregnancy and childbirth, to help expectant mothers manage discomfort, reduce stress, and improve their overall well-being.

Acupuncture provides numerous health benefits, including pain treatment, stress reduction, immune system support, and specialist care for women's health. Acupuncture's holistic approach, steeped in traditional Chinese medicine, offers a unique viewpoint on well-being, addressing both symptoms and underlying imbalances within the body. As research continues to elucidate the principles underlying acupuncture's success, its incorporation into mainstream healthcare is a promising option for improving general health and wellness.

CHAPTER 4
ACUPUNCTURE IN MODERN MEDICINE

Acupuncture has been widely integrated into modern medicine, particularly within the framework of integrative medicine techniques. In this environment, the emphasis is on integrating traditional methods with Western medicine to improve patient results.

One significant area where acupuncture has found application is in hospital settings. Hospitals are increasingly acknowledging acupuncture's potential benefits in the treatment of a variety of health issues. Integrating acupuncture into hospital settings provides patients with a more thorough and holistic approach to therapy. The practice is viewed as a supplemental therapy that can be used in conjunction with traditional medical treatments. This integration demonstrates a change toward a more patient-centered approach that recognizes the usefulness of various therapy methods.

Collaborations with Western medicine highlight the developing interaction between acupuncture and current medical treatments. Healthcare practitioners from traditional Chinese medicine (TCM) and Western medicine are increasingly working together to give patients a more comprehensive treatment plan. The combination of these two medical paradigms enables a more thorough understanding of health issues and a wider choice of treatment alternatives.

These collaborations seek to bridge the gap between Eastern and Western medical ideologies, resulting in a more inclusive and patient-centered healthcare system. As acupuncture becomes more widely accepted in Western medicine, the opportunity for joint initiatives to enhance patient outcomes grows.

<u>Scientific Research and Evidence:</u>

An increasing corpus of scientific study and data supports the use of acupuncture in modern medicine. Clinical studies are an essential component of this evidence base, enabling rigorous examinations of the efficacy of acupuncture in a variety of clinical situations. Acupuncture's effectiveness in comparison to mainstream medical procedures or placebo treatments can be established using rigorous study designs, such as randomized controlled trials (RCTs). These studies provide important insights into the precise illnesses for which acupuncture may be most effective, explaining its mechanisms of action and refining its application in modern healthcare settings.

Meta-analyses and reviews are critical in synthesizing the findings from various clinical trials, providing a thorough perspective of the available evidence. These studies critically assess the research's quality and consistency, assisting in determining acupuncture's overall efficacy across a wide range of medical settings. Meta-analyses give a more solid statistical foundation by aggregating data from multiple research, allowing for a better understanding of acupuncture's overall impact on patient outcomes. Reviews also help by providing expert insights on the strengths and limits of available evidence, assisting practitioners and policymakers in their decision-making processes.

Acupuncture integration into modern medicine is a comprehensive process that combines practical applications with evidence-based support. As hospitals include more acupuncture in their treatment programs and cooperation between traditional and Western medicine grows, patients will benefit from a more holistic and tailored approach to healthcare. The scientific research and evidence confirming acupuncture's efficacy, notably through well-designed clinical trials and detailed meta-analyses, reinforces its place in the current medical scene. As the conversation between ancient healing techniques and modern medicine continues, the possibility for improved patient care through the use of acupuncture grows.

CHAPTER 5
PREPARING FOR AN ACUPUNCTURE SESSION

Preparing for an acupuncture session is an important step in maximizing the potential benefits of this ancient Chinese medical treatment. Finding a qualified practitioner is the first and most important consideration in this procedure. Choosing a qualified and licensed acupuncturist guarantees that the therapy is safe and effective. A qualified practitioner often holds an acupuncture degree and has had considerable training, including hands-on experience with needling techniques, anatomy, and traditional Chinese medical concepts. Individuals might look for a qualified practitioner by consulting professional associations, or licensing boards, or asking healthcare providers for suggestions.

The initial consultation and assessment steps are critical in personalizing acupuncture therapy to each individual's distinct needs. During this stage, the acupuncturist does a thorough assessment, which may include a review of medical history, lifestyle factors, and a physical exam. This complete assessment helps to identify underlying abnormalities or obstructions in the body's energy flow, also known as Qi. To acquire a better understanding of the patient's condition, the acupuncturist may also use classical diagnostic methods including pulse and tongue diagnosis. This comprehensive evaluation results in an individualized treatment plan that targets specific acupuncture points to restore balance and promote general well-being.

Individuals considering or undergoing acupuncture should be aware of what to expect throughout the procedure. Acupuncture involves inserting thin, sterilized needles into particular acupuncture sites on the body. These sites are deliberately placed along meridians, which are conduits through which Qi moves. The insertion of needles is usually painless, with feelings ranging from tingling to minor discomfort. Once the needles are in place, the patient normally lies comfortably for a certain amount of time, usually 15 to 30 minutes. During this period, the acupuncturist may physically stimulate the needles or use other techniques to improve the therapeutic benefits, such as heat, electrical stimulation, or cupping. Individuals should discuss honestly with their acupuncturist about any sensations or pain they feel during the treatment.

Aftercare and follow-up are essential parts of the acupuncture procedure, contributing to the overall success of the treatment. Following an acupuncture session, people may have a variety of reactions, such as relaxation, improved energy, or a transient worsening of symptoms before improving. Patients must engage in adequate aftercare procedures to maximize the advantages and assist the body's healing processes. Hydration, rest, and avoiding vigorous activity immediately following a session are frequently advised. Furthermore, clients should adhere to any special advice given by the acupuncturist, such as food suggestions or self-care techniques. Regular follow-up appointments may be recommended to preserve the benefits of acupuncture and treat any lingering health issues.

This collaborative approach between the acupuncturist and the patient helps to ensure the long-term effectiveness of acupuncture as a holistic healthcare modality.

Preparing for an acupuncture session entails several interconnected principles that add to the effectiveness and safety of this traditional Chinese medicine treatment. Finding a qualified practitioner assures skill and adherence to professional standards, laying the groundwork for a successful acupuncture encounter. The initial consultation and assessment phase, which includes a thorough evaluation of the patient's history and condition, prepares the way for a unique treatment plan that addresses specific imbalances. Understanding what to expect during an acupuncture session promotes comfort and cooperation between the acupuncturist and the patient, resulting in open communication and a more effective therapeutic process. Finally, aftercare and follow-up are critical in maintaining the advantages of acupuncture, improving overall well-being, and treating any lingering health concerns. These ideas work together to create a comprehensive framework for those who want to get the most out of their acupuncture experience and maximize its potential for improving health and balance.

CHAPTER 6
SAFETY AND CONSIDERATIONS

Ensuring the safety of acupuncture techniques is critical in the practice of this ancient Chinese medical art. Acupuncture is the insertion of tiny needles into particular places on the body to enhance energy flow and healing. To avoid infections, using sterile needles is an important safety precaution. Practitioners must follow strict hygiene guidelines, including using single-use, disposable needles and keeping the clinic clean. Sterilization techniques are critical to reducing the danger of bacterial contamination and maintaining the patient's safety.

Another important safety factor is the acupuncturist's training and certification. Proper knowledge and expertise are required to comprehend the human anatomy, precisely locate acupuncture points, and identify potential issues. Licensed acupuncturists receive extensive training, frequently completing formal education programs and getting practical experience under supervision before practicing independently.

This guarantees that they have the skills required to conduct acupuncture safely, reducing the chance of adverse outcomes.

Furthermore, a thorough evaluation of the patient's medical history is critical in assuring safety during acupuncture sessions. Acupuncturists must be aware of any pre-existing medical issues, allergies, or drugs that could affect the therapy. Comprehensive intake questionnaires and extensive discussions allow practitioners to personalize their approach to each client, taking into consideration their specific health needs.

This tailored technique considerably improves the overall safety of acupuncture treatments.

<u>Contraindications and precautions:</u>

Understanding the contraindications and warnings of acupuncture is essential for offering safe and successful treatments. Certain conditions may render acupuncture ineffective or necessitate particular precautions to reduce dangers. Contraindications are conditions in which acupuncture should be avoided totally, whereas precautions are changes or close monitoring during treatment.

One major contraindication is the use of acupuncture during pregnancy, particularly at specific acupuncture points that may cause uterine contractions. To avoid causing injury to the growing fetus, acupuncturists should use caution and avoid particular sites or procedures. Similarly, people who have bleeding disorders or are taking anticoagulants may be more likely to experience bleeding or bruising at the needle insertion sites, making acupuncture inadvisable or demanding particular care.

Pre-existing medical disorders such as uncontrolled hypertension, epilepsy, or certain skin conditions may necessitate further care during acupuncture treatments. Practitioners must thoroughly assess the individual's health status and make informed decisions about the appropriateness of acupuncture in certain situations. Communication with other healthcare providers and participation with a patient's total healthcare team is critical for ensuring a thorough grasp of the patient's health and making informed decisions about acupuncture treatments.

Acupuncturists should also consider their patients' psychological well-being. Individuals who are afraid of needles, have significant anxiety, or have psychiatric disorders may not be good candidates for acupuncture, and they may require additional support and therapy to address their issues. An acupuncturist's role in providing safe and effective care includes being aware of contraindications and being able to alter treatment plans as needed.

Potential Side Effects:

While acupuncture is usually thought to be safe when conducted by skilled practitioners, it, like any other medical intervention, has the potential for negative effects.

Understanding and managing these adverse effects is critical to the patient's general well-being and the legitimacy of acupuncture as a therapeutic therapy.

One common adverse effect is minor soreness or bruising at the needle insertion sites.

This is usually temporary and resolves rapidly. Acupuncturists can reduce this danger by using thin needles, following good techniques, and taking into account the patient's sensitivity. Adequate communication with the patient about anticipated discomfort is critical for managing expectations and addressing any concerns they may have.

Some people may feel dizzy or lightheaded during or after receiving acupuncture. This can be ascribed to a variety of variables, including endorphin release, changes in blood pressure, and individual sensitivity. Practitioners must be watchful during treatments, ensuring that patients are comfortably positioned and ready to make modifications as necessary. Adequate post-treatment advice, such as urging patients to rise slowly and avoid rapid movements, can help to reduce this adverse effect.

In rare situations, more significant consequences, such as infections or organ damage, may occur. These cases are usually related to poor hygiene, inaccurate needling practices, or insufficient training. Strict attention to safety precautions, such as using sterilized needles and receiving sufficient training, dramatically minimizes the incidence of such consequences. To maintain the greatest levels of safety and patient care, acupuncturists must be aware of potential hazards, constantly update their expertise, and respond quickly to any adverse events that arise.

Acupuncture is a treatment method with a long history and numerous potential advantages. However, guaranteeing the safety of acupuncture operations necessitates a thorough study and application of safety precautions and contraindications, as well as awareness of potential side effects. Acupuncturists who follow these principles can deliver successful and safe treatments, contributing to their patients' general well-being and encouraging the continued acceptance of acupuncture as a complementary and alternative medicine.

CHAPTER 7
EXPLORING TRADITIONAL CHINESE MEDICINE

TCM is a holistic healing method that has been practiced for hundreds of years and is based on ancient Chinese philosophy and culture. Acupuncture is a popular and well-known treatment among the several modalities found in TCM. Acupuncture is the insertion of tiny needles into particular places on the body to promote energy flow and restore equilibrium. This ancient practice is based on the concept of Qi or vital energy that travels through the body via meridians.

Understanding the benefits and procedures of acupuncture necessitates diving into its extensive history and concepts.

<u>Acupuncture benefits:</u>

Acupuncture is known for its wide variety of therapeutic advantages. One significant advantage is its efficacy in pain treatment. Acupuncture has been shown in numerous trials to effectively treat chronic pain disorders such as back pain, osteoarthritis, and migraines.

Endorphin release and nervous system modification are thought to be the mechanisms underlying this analgesic action. Acupuncture has also shown potential in lowering stress and anxiety, increase relaxation, and enhancing sleep quality.

Its holistic approach to wellness includes improving immune function, controlling hormone imbalances, and promoting mental health.

<u>Acupuncture techniques:</u>

Acupuncture treatments are based on traditional Chinese medicine and Qi manipulation. Meridians, which are the body's energy lines, are stimulated by placing needles into certain acupuncture spots. The selection of locations and the depth of needle insertion are determined by the patient's condition and the desired therapeutic outcome.

Manual manipulation of the needles, electroacupuncture, which includes passing a low electric current through the needles, and moxibustion, which involves burning dried mugwort near the skin to warm and energize the Qi. Understanding these strategies allows practitioners to personalize therapies to specific needs and circumstances.

Exploring Traditional Chinese Medicine.

<u>Herbal Medicines:</u>

In addition to acupuncture, herbal medicine is an important aspect of TCM. It involves the use of plant-based components such as roots, leaves, and seeds to treat a variety of health problems. Ginseng, licorice root, astragalus, and ginger are among the most commonly utilized herbs in TCM.

These herbs are picked for their particular qualities, flavors, and therapeutic effects. The combining of herbs into formulations is an important part of TCM herbal therapy, as numerous ingredients work together to balance the body's Qi and address the underlying cause of imbalances.

Herbal formulas:

TCM practitioners provide herbal formulae that are suited to a person's specific constitution and health situation.

These formulae frequently include a combination of primary herbs, which target the major symptoms or imbalances, and secondary herbs, which supplement the primary herbs or address secondary symptoms. The technique of compounding herbs necessitates a thorough understanding of TCM principles, diagnosis, and each herb's unique qualities.

Herbal formulations are often administered as decoctions, powders, tablets, or tinctures.

This individualized approach enables TCM practitioners to treat a wide range of health issues and enhance general well-being.

Exploring Traditional Chinese Medicine.

<u>Tai Chi and Qigong:</u>

Tai Chi and Qi Gong are mind-body techniques with roots in ancient Chinese philosophy.

These smooth, flowing motions aim to cultivate and balance the body's Qi, encouraging health and energy. Tai Chi is a martial technique that incorporates slow, deliberate motions, controlled breathing, and meditation. Qi Gong, on the other hand, refers to a broader spectrum of activities such as breath control, meditation, and movement. Both activities aim to improve the flow of Qi and promote general health and well-being.

<u>Mind/Body Practices:</u>

Tai Chi and Qi Gong both emphasize the importance of the mind-body connection. Practitioners are advised to create a state of mindfulness, in which the mind is completely engaged in the present moment. This mental focus, combined with deliberate movements and controlled breathing, aids in stress reduction, attention, and mental clarity. Regular Tai Chi and Qi Gong practice has been linked to several health advantages, including enhanced balance, flexibility, and cardiovascular health. These mind-body practices are suitable for people of all ages and fitness levels, making them effective instruments for improving holistic wellness.

<u>Complementary Techniques:</u>

Tai Chi and Qi Gong are often used as complementing methods in holistic wellness programs.

When paired with acupuncture and herbal treatment, these activities improve the overall effectiveness of TCM. For example, including Tai Chi in a chronic pain treatment regimen helps increase mobility and reduce stiffness. Qi Gong's emphasis on breath control and meditation compliments acupuncture's relaxing benefits, making it an excellent supplement for stress management and mental wellness. Integrating these complimentary strategies enables TCM practitioners to provide a more comprehensive approach to patient care, addressing physical, mental, and energetic components of health.

CONCLUSION

The study of acupuncture in the context of Traditional Chinese Medicine reveals a comprehensive and holistic approach to health and wellness.

Acupuncture, which originated in ancient Chinese philosophy and the notion of Qi, provides a wide range of therapeutic advantages. Acupuncture is a multifaceted treatment that addresses the interconnectivity of the body, mind, and spirit.

Acupuncture procedures, such as needle insertion, manual manipulation, electroacupuncture, and moxibustion, are based on TCM principles. Understanding meridians, acupuncture sites, and the tailored selection of procedures enables practitioners to tailor treatments to specific illnesses and restore equilibrium within the body's energy system.

Aside from acupuncture, Traditional Chinese Medicine includes herbal medicine, which involves the use of various plant-based compounds in carefully crafted combinations to treat a wide range of health concerns.

The tailored approach to herbal formulations emphasizes the significance of understanding TCM principles, herbal qualities, and individual diagnosis.

Tai Chi and Qi Gong, as mind-body practices, help to promote Qi cultivation and balance, which contributes to TCM's holistic approach.

These practices, which emphasize intentional movements, controlled breathing, and mindfulness, provide additional opportunities for improving physical, mental, and energy well-being. When Tai Chi and Qi Gong are combined with complete wellness programs, they complement acupuncture and herbal therapy, resulting in a more holistic approach to patient care.

In essence, acupuncture's benefits and practices, as well as its integration with other modalities of Traditional Chinese Medicine, provide a comprehensive framework for understanding and treating health.

This ancient system, with its emphasis on balance, harmony, and personalized care, continues to contribute to the changing landscape of complementary and alternative medicine by providing a unique viewpoint on improving well-being and preventing sickness.